INTERMITTENT FASTING FOR WOMEN OVER 40

A Concise Guide to restarting metabolism and boosting energy

Willie S. Harper

OTHER BOOKS BY THE AUTHOR

HASHIMOTO DIET FOR NEWLY DIAGNOSED RECIPE COOKBOOK

NO GALLBLADDER DIET RECIPE COOKBOOK

INSULIN RESISTANCE DIET COOKBOOK

PLANT BASED MEDITERRANEAN DIET COOKBOOK

JUICING FOR CANCER RECIPE BOOK FOR NEWLY DIAGNOSED

JUICING FOR DIABETES RECIPE BOOK

ALZHEIMER'S SOLUTION DIET COOKBOOK FOR BEGINNERS

DIVERTICULITIS DIET COOKBOOK

ACID REFLUX DIET COOKBOOK FOR BEGINNERS

AYURVEDA COOKBOOK FOR WOMEN

LOW OXALATE DIET BOOK

BARIATRIC DIET COOKBOOK

JUICING RECIPES FOR GUT HEALTH

AFIB COOKBOOK

THE AUTOIMMUNE PROTOCOL COOKBOOK

HEART HEALTHY COOKBOOK FOR BEGINNERS 2023

GOUT DIET COOKBOOK

RENAL DIET SMOOTHIE RECIPES FOR SENIORS

DIABETIC RENAL DIET COOKBOOK

CIRRHOSIS DIET CONTROL COOKBOOK

TABLE OF CONTENT

Introduction

Living in a tiny village tucked away among rolling hills, Alice was a cheerful woman. She was a woman in her early forties who was always trying to become healthier and better for her health. When she was perusing a neighbouring bookshop one day, she became intrigued by a book called "Intermittent Fasting for Women over 40". Her curiosity was piqued, and she couldn't resist the allure of its intriguing contents.

As Alice turned the pages, a gripping story came into view. It described the life of Emily, a made-up woman who had started an intermittent fasting adventure. When Emily experienced an increase in energy, mental clarity, and a healthier relationship with food, her life was forever altered. She glowed brighter, had more self-assurance, and lost weight.

In Emily's story, Alice saw a reflection of herself that inspired her to envision a new iteration of herself. The book provided her with a personalized road map by emphasizing the most effective fasting routines, overcoming challenges, and the need for self-care.

Alice was overcome with optimism and a sensation of newfound power as she closed the book. She embarked on her intermittent fasting adventure armed with knowledge, eager to find the hidden energy and health treasures that lay ahead of her on this life-altering path.

Chapter 1: Understanding Intermittent Fasting

Due to its purported health benefits, the age-old practice of intermittent fasting has attracted a lot of attention recently. Fundamentally, intermittent fasting involves alternating between eating and fasting periods. But it has effects on the body that go beyond calorie restriction alone, even at the molecular level.

Understanding intermittent fasting requires an understanding of the underlying workings of our biological process. Our bodies begin a multitude of metabolic processes to digest and utilize nutrients when we eat. When fasting, the body uses the fat and glycogen that have been collected as energy stores.

In addition to helping people lose weight, intermittent fasting offers numerous other advantages. It has shown potential in promoting cellular regeneration and repair, promoting heart health, and raising insulin sensitivity. Furthermore, a number of studies suggest that intermittent fasting may improve longevity and brain function.

Two examples of intermittent fasting methods include the 16/8 approach (fasting for 16 hours and eating within an 8-hour window) and alternate-day fasting. Each method is adaptable, allowing users to pick the one that most closely matches their requirements and goals.

With awareness of the evidence supporting intermittent fasting, people may profit from its potential advantages and decide whether to incorporate it into their lives.

Chapter 2: Tailoring Intermittent Fasting to Women Over 40

It is crucial to adjust intermittent fasting to the particular requirements of women over 40 in order to maximize its advantages and take into account the distinctive physiological changes that take place at this stage of life. Intermittent fasting must be done with consideration for hormonal changes, metabolic changes, and general well-being.

Hormonal changes in women over 40, such as perimenopause and menopause, are common and can affect metabolism and body composition. As a result, it's critical to modify your fasting plans properly. Greater support for general hormonal health can be provided by shorter fasting intervals or a progressive move to longer fasts.

When designing intermittent fasting, it is crucial to take women's health into account. To guarantee that vital vitamins, minerals, and macronutrients are absorbed, it is essential to consume enough nutrition and to pay attention to nourishing foods. For overall health, it is also crucial to address any specific health issues or nutritional deficiencies, promote bone health with adequate calcium, and get enough vitamin D.

Additionally, intermittent fasting variations that fit their lifestyle and tastes may be advantageous for women over 40. Flexible fasting schedules can still reap the benefits of intermittent fastings, such as time-restricted eating or alternate-day fasting.

Individuals can maximize metabolic health, hormone balance, and general wellness by adopting intermittent fasting to the specific requirements of women over 40, releasing the full potential of this effective practice for this particular stage of life.

Chapter 3: Getting Started

For women over 40, beginning an intermittent fasting regimen can be a thrilling and empowering experience. The following are some necessary actions to start down this road:

1. Establish Specific Objectives: Explain why you choose to practice intermittent fasting. Having a defined purpose will help you stay on track throughout the process, whether it's weight management, increased energy, or general wellness.

2. Select the Appropriate Fasting Schedule: Research several fasting practices and pick one that fits your lifestyle and interests. Popular choices include the 16/8 approach, which involves fasting for 16 hours and eating within an 8-hour window, and the 5:2 method, which involves eating normally for 5 days and restricting calories for 2 days that are not consecutive.

3. Begin Gradually: If you're new to intermittent fasting, you might want to take it slowly at first. Start with shorter fasting windows and then progressively lengthen them as you get more accustomed to the fasting schedule.

4. Make a Meal Plan. Focus on complete, nutrient-dense meals when making your meal plan. To ensure you satisfy your nutritional needs, give lean proteins, healthy fats, fruits, vegetables, and complex carbohydrates priority during your meal window.

5. Maintain Proper Hydration: When fasting, maintaining proper hydration is essential. To enhance digestion, energy levels, and general well-being, drink lots of water throughout the day.

6. Practice Mindful Meal: During your meal window, pay attention to your body's signals of hunger and fullness. To savor and appreciate your meals while encouraging a positive relationship with food, engage in mindful eating.

7. Track Your Progress: Record your eating and fasting routines as well as any adjustments you make to your energy, mood, or weight. By doing so, you may evaluate what suits you the best and make any required adjustments.

8. Seek Support: Participate in an encouraging environment, join discussion boards online, or ask a certified dietitian or healthcare provider with expertise in intermittent fasting for

advice. Having a support network can offer inspiration, reassurance, and tailored guidance.

Every person is different, so pay attention to your body and modify your fasting strategy as necessary. Starting an intermittent fasting regimen can be a life-changing experience for women over 40 who are looking to improve their health and general well-being.

Chapter 4: Navigating Challenges

To overcome the challenges encountered on the intermittent fasting journey for women over 40, resilience and adaptation are required. Even while the trip may not always be simple, real growth and transformation are only possible via overcoming these challenges.

One of the most common issues is the continual presence of hunger and cravings. As the body becomes adjusted to the new eating patterns, it may begin to resist strong signals that it needs sustenance. It is essential to remember during these times the long-term advantages of intermittent fasting. Remind yourself that any slight discomfort is nothing compared to the potential benefits, stay hydrated, and focus on fun activities.

Food-related social activities and gatherings can occasionally be challenging. Peer pressure and the desire to indulge can make even the most steadfast people give in. But don't worry—there are effective strategies to deal with these situations. Modify your fasting schedule or eating window in advance of the event. Talk to your loved ones about your dietary choices, focusing on your connections and shared experiences rather than just the food.

There can be a plateau along the way where it seems like your efforts aren't moving the needle. These are the occasions when ambiguity may begin to creep in, raising questions about the effectiveness of intermittent fasting.

Accept the opportunity for reflection and improvement, though. Consult with experts, alter your fasting schedule, or adopt novel techniques like exercise or mindful eating. You can go past plateaus and onto the next level with perseverance.

Never forget that challenges are opportunities for growth and resilience rather than obstacles. Accept them as necessary obstacles on the way, knowing that each one you overcome will bring you closer to your goals.

Keep your attention on the task at hand, make appropriate adjustments, and celebrate each success. The challenges you have while adhering to the intermittent fasting diet are not barriers; rather, they are stepping stones that will eventually assist you in becoming a healthier, happier, and more self-assured version of yourself.

Chapter 5: 7 DAY MEALPLAN

Here's a sample 7-day meal plan suitable for intermittent fasting for women over 40. This plan incorporates nutritious and balanced meals within the designated eating window:

Day 1:

- Eating Window: 12:00 PM - 8:00 PM

- Lunch: Grilled chicken breast with mixed greens, cherry tomatoes, cucumber, and balsamic vinaigrette.

- Snack: Greek yogurt with a handful of almonds.

- Dinner: Baked salmon with roasted asparagus and quinoa.

- Snack: Sliced apple with almond butter.

Day 2:

- Eating Window: 1:00 PM - 9:00 PM

- Lunch: Quinoa salad with grilled vegetables, chickpeas, and lemon-tahini dressing.

- Snack: Carrot sticks with hummus.

- Dinner: Grilled tofu with stir-fried broccoli, bell peppers, and brown rice.

- Snack: Mixed berries with a dollop of Greek yogurt.

Day 3:

- Eating Window: 11:00 AM - 7:00 PM

- Lunch: Spinach and feta omelet with a side of whole wheat toast.

- Snack: Celery sticks with almond butter.

- Dinner: Grilled shrimp skewers with roasted zucchini and cauliflower rice.

- Snack: Dark chocolate square.

Day 4:

- Eating Window: 12:00 PM - 8:00 PM

- Lunch: Quinoa and black bean salad with cherry tomatoes, avocado, and lime-cilantro dressing.

- Snack: Hard-boiled egg.

- Dinner: Grilled chicken with steamed broccoli and sweet potato wedges.

- Snack: Sliced cucumber with tzatziki dip.

Day 5:

- Eating Window: 1:00 PM - 9:00 PM

- Lunch: Mediterranean salad with mixed greens, olives, feta cheese, cherry tomatoes, and lemon vinaigrette.

- Snack: Mixed nuts.

- Dinner: Baked cod with roasted Brussels sprouts and quinoa.

- Snack: Berries with a dollop of coconut yogurt.

Day 6:

- Eating Window: 11:00 AM - 7:00 PM

- Lunch: Lentil soup with a side of mixed green salad.

- Snack: Cottage cheese with sliced peaches.

- Dinner: Grilled steak with roasted asparagus and sweet potato mash.

- Snack: Rice cake with almond butter.

Day 7:

- Eating Window: 12:00 PM - 8:00 PM

- Lunch: Quinoa and roasted vegetable wrap with hummus.

- Snack: Veggie sticks with guacamole.

- Dinner: Baked chicken breast with sautéed spinach and cauliflower rice.

- Snack: Yogurt with mixed berries and a sprinkle of granola.

Remember to adjust the portion sizes based on your individual needs and preferences. Additionally, ensure that you stay hydrated throughout the day by drinking plenty of water. This meal plan serves as a starting point and can be customized to suit your specific dietary requirements and taste preferences.

Chapter 6: Supporting Your Journey

For a woman over 40 to start the intermittent fasting journey, more is required than just a diet plan and fasting schedule. It needs a thorough plan that takes into account every aspect of your life. The tactics listed below will facilitate your journey and ensure long-term success:

1. Educate Yourself: Take some time to read up on the concepts and research behind intermittent fasting. Recognize its impacts on your body and any benefits it might offer. This knowledge can help you make sensible decisions and keep your motivation high while traveling.

Make self-care a priority. Intermittent fasting requires self-care to maintain overall well-being. Get enough sleep, manage your stress, engage in interesting hobbies, and set aside time for relaxation. Your ability to think positively and accomplish long-lasting progress depends on maintaining strong physical and mental health.

3. Maintain Proper Hydration: It's crucial to maintain proper hydration all day long and during fasting. Drink enough water to support metabolism, digestion, and overall health. You can also add herbal teas or infusions to increase flavor and variety.

4. Move Your Body: Make regular exercise a part of your daily schedule. Find exercises you enjoy doing, such as jogging, yoga, or weight training. Exercise boosts a person's energy levels, happiness, and overall well-being while also assisting with weight management.

5. Seek Support: Surround yourself with a group of people who agree with you, whether they be friends, family, or other acquaintances. Discuss your experience, seek guidance as needed, and share your journey. Having a support network during difficult times can provide motivation, responsibility, and drive.

6. Track Your Progress: Keep a journal of the times you fast, your meals, and any changes you see. This makes it possible for you to keep track of your progress, identify trends, and make adjustments as needed. Celebrate both little and big victories to keep yourself motivated and devoted to your goals.

There is no one-size-fits-all approach to intermittent fasting, so be adaptable and flexible. Be prepared to adjust your fasting schedule, diet plan, or methods to suit your body's needs. Pay attention to your body and make any necessary adjustments if you want to make a sustainable development.

8. Celebrate Successes Outside of the Scale: Although losing weight may be a goal, success shouldn't solely be based on the reading on the scale. Celebrate additional achievements such as higher energy, better sleep, increased mental clarity, or an improved mood. These triumphs off the scale serve as equally important indicators of your growth.

Remember that your experience with IF is unique to you. Accept the process, be kind to yourself, and consider setbacks as opportunities to grow. By offering thorough support for your journey, you can establish a fulfilling lifestyle that supports general health, well-being, and long-term success.

Chapter 7: Monitoring and Adjusting

It's crucial to track your progress and make adjustments to your intermittent fasting plan if you want to stay on track and reach your goals. Take into account the following crucial tactics to help you correctly monitor and make the required adjustments:

1. Keep a Fasting Log: Record when you fast, when you eat, and any noteworthy observations or mood changes. This journal will help you identify patterns and trends in your fasting schedule and will provide you with valuable information about it.

2. Track Your Food Consumption: Consider using a food diary or smartphone app to keep tabs on your meals and calorie intake during your eating window. You will be better able to comprehend your nutritional consumption and be able to make any necessary adjustments as a result.

3. Pay Attention to Your Body: Pay special attention to how you feel both during and after fasting periods. Keep an eye on your energy level, appetite, and overall wellness. If you frequently experience excessive hunger or low energy, it

may be necessary to adjust your fasting schedule or the composition of your meals.

4. Modify Your Fasting Plan: If you find that your current fasting plan isn't working for you, be willing to adjust it. To determine which fasting window suits your body and way of life the best, experiment with ones that are shorter or longer in duration. It could take some trial and error, so be patient and pay close attention to how your body responds.

5. Modify the Nutrient Content of Your Meals: Assess Your Meals' Nutrient Content and Make Modifications as Necessary. Make sure your diet is well-balanced with an assortment of fruits and vegetables, excellent fats, and enough protein. Modify portion sizes and macronutrient ratios to meet your health and weight loss goals.

6. Consult a professional: If you require guidance on how to monitor or adjust your intermittent fasting approach from a registered dietitian or other healthcare professionals, seek it out. They can provide customized guidance based on your unique needs and help you get over any challenges you might encounter.

7. Constantly Reevaluate Your Goals: Set aside time to review and reevaluate your goals regularly. Are they still in keeping with your overall health and well-being objectives? You might need to adjust your objectives or make new ones to maintain your motivation and involvement in the process.

Keep in mind that monitoring and adjusting are continual processes as your body and lifestyle change. Be mindful of the signs your body sends and be open to adjusting your approach when engaging in intermittent fasting if you want to ensure a lasting and satisfying experience.

Chapter 8: FAQs about Intermittent Fasting

How does intermittent fasting work?

A practice of eating called intermittent fasting alternates between periods of fasting and eating. It concentrates on when you eat rather than what you consume. The 16/8 approach (fasting for 16 hours and eating within an 8-hour window) and the 5:2 strategy (eating normally for 5 days and restricting calories on 2 separate days) are two popular fasting strategies.

Is intermittent fasting appropriate for women over the age of 40?

Yes, women over 40 can benefit from intermittent fasting. It's crucial to approach it cautiously and take into account each person's unique health situation. To make sure it fits your unique needs and any pre-existing medical issues, it is advised that you consult with a healthcare practitioner or certified dietitian.

Will intermittent fasting aid in the loss of weight?

Intermittent fasting can be a useful weight-loss method. A calorie deficit and fat burning may be facilitated by limiting the eating window. For lasting weight loss, it's crucial to keep up a balanced diet and keep an eye on overall calorie consumption during the eating window.

Can I consume liquids when I'm fasting?

You can drink non-caloric liquids during fasting periods, including water, herbal tea, and black coffee. These drinks may aid in appetite suppression and can help you stay hydrated.

Can I work out while I'm fasting?

In general, it is okay to exercise when fasting. However, it's crucial to pay attention to your body and change the time and intensity of your workouts as necessary. To ensure they have enough energy and nutrition for their activity, some people might prefer to exercise within the eating window.

Do intermittent fasting's potential negative effects exist?

Although most people find intermittent fasting to be harmless, some people may have adverse effects like hunger, irritation, or trouble concentrating. These adverse effects typically pass quickly as the body acclimates. Consult a healthcare provider if you have any worries or encounter persistent bad symptoms.

Can I still use my meds and dietary supplements while fasting?

It's crucial to adhere to your healthcare provider's recommendations for taking supplements and medications during fasting times. For particular advice, speak with your healthcare professional since some drugs may need to be taken with food.

How long does it take for intermittent fasting to produce results?

Individual characteristics, like body composition, metabolism, and adherence to the fasting regimen, can affect results. While some people may notice changes within a few weeks, others might not. Patience and consistency are crucial for getting the desired results.

Please keep in mind that while these FAQs offer broad information, specific facts may vary. Before beginning intermittent fasting or making other significant dietary or lifestyle changes, it is advised that you speak with a healthcare provider or qualified dietitian.

Conclusion

In this book, developed specifically for women over 40, the topic of intermittent fasting has been explored. You have received insightful knowledge, practical suggestions, and tactics to support you in your intermittent fasting journey.

Understanding the principles of intermittent fasting, customizing it to meet your unique needs, and putting the suggested meal plans and procedures into practice can help you reap the benefits of this eating pattern. A happier and more powerful existence is possible with intermittent fasting, which also helps with weight management, improved metabolic health, and overall well-being.

Throughout this book, we have discussed the challenges, responded to numerous questions, and offered practical guidance for monitoring and adjusting your strategy. Remember that intermittent fasting is a personal journey that may take some testing and adaptation to discover what works best for you.

As you continue on this transforming journey, practice patience, self-kindness, and openness. Keep working toward your goals, pay attention to your body's signals, and ask for assistance when you need it. If you are dedicated and diligent, you can discover the various benefits that intermittent fasting can offer.

As you set out on your road to an intermittent fasting lifestyle that is healthier and happier for you, may this book be your trustworthy guide. Accept the journey, celebrate your successes, and look ahead to a time when your health and happiness are at their peak.